Contents

Some words are printed in bold, **like this**. You can find out what they mean in the glossary.

Finding out about behaviour

What is behaviour?

Have you ever wondered why people behave the way they do? Some people always seem happy and content, while others are full of anger and **aggression**. Some people take drugs, drink too much alcohol, or eat so much that they become **obese**. There are people who love to exercise, and people who never move away from their television or computer screen.

The world around you is changing all the time and the way you behave changes in response to your environment. The way people behave affects how they feel, and it also affects their health.

If you watch animals – your pets or animals in the wild – you will see that they have clear patterns of behaviour. They react to hunger and they respond to meeting other animals. In other words, they react to the world around them. In this book you will look at how the science you study in school can help you understand the way people and animals behave. You will find out how behaviour affects health.

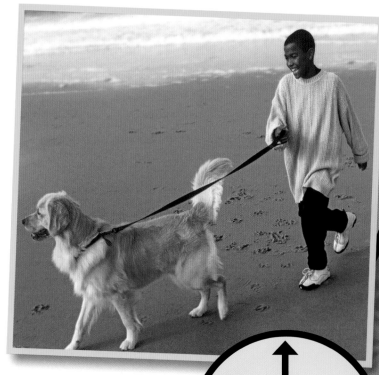

In scientific terms, behaviour is defined as: The actions displayed by an organism in response to its environment. The scientific study of animal behaviour is called **ethology**. Investigating animal behaviour can happen in many different places such as a laboratory, a zoological park, or the natural environment, from the depths of a rainforest to a deserted piece of waste ground.

Humans and other animals behave very differently. Scientists can learn a lot by studying both!

Leabharlanna Poiblí Chathair Bhaile Átha Cliath
Dublin City Public Libraries

Why Science Matters

Understanding Health and Behaviour

Ann Fullick

www.heinemannlibrary.co.uk
Visit our website to find out more information about Heinemann Library books.

To order:
☎ Phone +44 (0) 1865 888066
🗎 Fax +44 (0) 1865 314091
🖥 Visit www.heinemannlibrary.co.uk

Heinemann Library is an imprint of **Capstone Global Library Limited**, a company incorporated in England and Wales having its registered office at 7 Pilgrim Street, London, EC4V 6LB – Registered company number: 6695582

Heinemann is a registered trademark of Pearson Education Limited, under licence to Capstone Global Library Limited

Edited by Andrew Farrow, Megan Cotugno, and Harriet Milles
Designed by Steven Mead and Q2A Creative Solutions
Original illustrations © Pearson Education Limited
Illustrated by Gordon Hurden
Picture research by Ruth Blair
Produced by Alison Parsons
Originated by Heinemann Library
Printed and bound in China by Leo Paper Products

ISBN 978 0 431 04071 4 (hardback)
12 11 10 09 08
10 9 8 7 6 5 4 3 2 1

ISBN 978 0 431 04084 4 (paperback)
13 12 11 10 09
10 9 8 7 6 5 4 3 2 1

British Library Cataloguing in Publication data
Fullick, Ann, 1956-
Understanding health and behaviour. - (Why science matters)
613
A full catalogue record for this book is available from the British Library.

Acknowledgements
We would like to thank the following for permission to reproduce photographs: © Alamy pp 11 (Wolfgang Kaehler), 13 (Steve Bloom Images), 22 (tbkmedia.de), 26 (Profimedia International s.r.o.), 31 (ImageState), 35 (Mike Goldwater), 35 (Christa Knijff), 38 (Megapress), 44 (Trevor Smith); © Barcroft Media p 47; © Corbis pp 14 (Creasource), 17 (Roy Morsch), 18 (L. Clarke), 49 (David P Hall); © Corbis/Zefa pp 27 (Gary Salter), 40 (Mika), 42 (Mika); © Digital Vision p 23; © FLPA/Konrad Wothe; Miden Pictures p 23; © Getty Images pp 4 (Lars Klove Photo Service), 25 (Justin Sullivan), 29 (Nick White); © istockphoto.com p 23; © Nature Picture Library p 20 (Pete Oxford); © Photolibrary/Oxford Scientific/TC Nature p 33; © Photolibrary/Phototake Science/Collection CNRI p 36; © Science Photo Library pp 5, 7 (Wellcome Dept. of Imaging Neuroscience), 12 (Photo Researchers), 48 (BSIP VEM). Background images supplied by ©istockphoto.

Cover image of an MRI brain scan reproduced with permission of © Getty Images/Photodisc. Background design reproduced with permission of ©istockphoto.

We would like to thank Michael J. Reiss for his invaluable assistance in the preparation of this book.

Every effort has been made to contact copyright holders of any material reproduced in this book. Any omissions will be rectified in subsequent printings if notice is given to the publishers.

Disclaimer
All the Internet addresses (URLs) given in this book were valid at the time of going to press. However, due to the dynamic nature of the Internet, some addresses may have changed, or sites may have ceased to exist since publication. While the author and publishers regret any inconvenience this may cause readers, no responsibility for any such changes can be accepted by either the author or the publishers.

Studying human behaviour can be easier than studying other animals because people can explain what they are doing and why. However, studying human behaviour is full of difficulties and raises lots of **ethical issues**. For example, it is not ethical to force humans to behave in a particular way for an experiment.

Lorenz and Tinbergen – the fathers of ethology

Scientists have observed animal behaviour for many years. However, it was the work of Austrian biologist Konrad Lorenz and Dutch biologist Nikolaas (Niko) Tinbergen in the 1930s–60s that really developed the science of ethology.

Lorenz developed many theories about how animal behaviour patterns develop, and the importance of **instinct**. Tinbergen produced evidence that supported Lorenz's ideas. Together they changed the way that animal behaviour was studied. Lorenz's most famous work was with geese. He observed that shortly after hatching, goslings follow their mother everywhere. Lorenz showed that this is due to an instinctive behaviour called imprinting. The goslings follow anything that moves and makes goose-like sounds. In the course of his research, Lorenz had many goslings imprinted on him (see photo above)! In 1973, Lorenz and Tinbergen were awarded the Nobel Prize in Physiology or Medicine for their work.

Responding to the environment

When you walk past a baker's shop it is very tempting to buy – and eat – a cake or doughnut. When a male dog walks past a lamp-post, he will sniff and urinate if given a chance. When the seasons change, birds take off and migrate to other countries, sometimes thousands of kilometres away. These examples of behaviour are all responses to a change in the environment. How do we recognize that our surroundings have changed?

Sensitivity

All animals have some degree of **sensitivity**. Many animals have well-developed **sense organs**, which respond to changes in the world around them.

- Eyes respond to light, which makes it possible to see changes taking place. For example, someone may see a display of delicious cakes when passing a bakery.
- Ears are sensitive to sounds, making it possible to communicate with others and hear changes in the environment such as an approaching car.
- The nose provides a sense of smell, which is particularly important to other animals such as dogs. A lamp-post carries hundreds of scent messages about other dogs that have visited the same place.
- Taste buds on the tongue provide a sense of taste, telling you if food is pleasant or not.
- Touch sensors in the skin provide information about the feel of the surroundings, for example whether a surface is soft, smooth, or prickly.

Different areas of the body have different numbers of sensory nerve endings. In this illustration, the enlarged areas of the body have a large number of sensory nerve endings. Sensory nerves send information about the world around you to the central nervous system. Then motor nerves carry the messages to the muscles, so you can act on that information.

The sense organs send electrical messages known as **nerve impulses** to the central nervous system. Depending on the type of animal, the central nervous system ranges from a simple tube to the complex brain and spinal cord of human beings. The information from the sense organs is sorted in the brain. Next, more impulses are sent out to stimulate the muscles of the body to move and respond.

Empathy

Pain

The human brain is very complicated but scientists are learning more and more about how it works from scans like these.

CUTTING EDGE: WATCHING THE BRAIN IN ACTION

MRI scanners allow researchers to see what is happening in the brains of animals, including humans. The scanners show which parts of the brain are active as we behave in different ways. A team of researchers from the United States have shown that when people feel rejected, the response in their brain is the same as though they were being physically hurt. It seems likely that this affects our behaviour and makes us try to look after the people who are close to us.

The brain

The human brain is organized into different areas. Each area deals with different information and helps control the behaviour of the body. The brain has some areas that control behaviour without any conscious thought on your part. Other areas involve conscious thought, which allows you to have control over how you behave. Scientists still have a great deal to learn about the interactions between the brain and behaviour.

Reflexes and simple behaviour

If you put your hand on something hot or sharp, you pull it away before even thinking about it. This response is a reflex. Reflex actions are the basis of a lot of animal behaviour. In humans, reflexes help keep you out of danger. They also control many of the basic functions of life such as breathing and the contractions of your gut muscles. It would be very hard work if you had to remember to breathe every few seconds, and consciously make your gut squeeze the food through your body!

THE SCIENCE YOU LEARN: REFLEX ARCS

In a reflex, a **stimulus** is picked up by the sensory receptors. The nerve impulse travels through a sensory nerve to the central nervous system. It then travels through a "short cut" straight back into the motor nerves. It travels on to the muscles, which contract and make your body react. This arrangement of nerves is called a reflex arc. Impulses also go up to your brain, so you know what has happened.

A reflex arc is a very rapid response to a change in the environment. It uses a reflective arc, which does not involve conscious thought.

① Sensory receptor (sensitive to heat)

② The sensory neurone carries the message to the CNS.

Spinal cord (CNS)

⑤ The effector organ (in this case a muscle) moves the hand away from the heat.

③ The relay neurone transfers the message to the motor neurone.

④ The motor neurone carries the message to the effector organ.

Conditioned reflexes and learning

Reflexes like blinking are not learned. Instead, they are present from birth. Many other reflexes are learned, often without us realizing. These are called **conditioned reflexes**. For example, when a baby learns to walk it has to think about every step. Watch a small child walking. It is obvious that they have to concentrate on moving their legs, using their arms to balance and thinking about where to put their feet. Then watch older children or adults walking around. The action has become completely reflex and there is no conscious thought involved at all.

If you have ever had a pet, from a dog to a goldfish, you will know that you can use external cues (signals) to change their behaviour. In other words, they can learn. When your dog sees you pick up the lead (the cue), he knows it is time for a walk and gets excited. When you touch the surface of the water a goldfish knows it is time to be fed and comes to the top of the tank. This learning is often the result of developing conditioned reflexes.

CASE STUDY

Pavlov and his dogs

In the late 19th and early 20th century, Russian scientist Ivan Pavlov set up a series of experiments with dogs. He showed that when dogs see their food, they start to produce saliva. Pavlov started ringing a bell just before he brought food to the dogs. In a short time the dogs would produce saliva when they heard the bell ring, without seeing or smelling their food. They had learnt to associate the bell with food, an example of learning through a conditioned reflex.

What drives behaviour?

There are certain basic needs that drive behaviour in all animals, from prawns to humans. One of the most fundamental drives is for food. Hunger is behind many different levels of behaviour. For example, carnivores eat other animals, so they have to catch their food. The behaviour involved in catching food varies enormously. The larvae of ant lions dig circular pits in soil and then hide themselves at the bottom of the pits. When insects fall into the pits, the ant lion pounces and devours its prey. This hunting behaviour is an instinct, which means that it is inherited behaviour that is pre-programmed and does not need to be learned. All members of a species show the same pattern of instinctive behaviour.

Lions – social hunters

African lions are social hunters. They work together as a team to surround and chase their prey. One lioness takes over from another until one is successful in bringing the prey down. Lion cubs have to learn how to hunt successfully. They have a number of instinctive behaviour patterns that help. Cubs, like domestic kittens, pounce on moving things. They flatten themselves with their bodies low to the ground and creep up on their siblings (brothers and sisters). However, they need to watch the adults and learn how to interact to become part of a hunting pride (group).

Sand with your sweet potato?

Some animal feeding behaviour is almost human. Scientists observed an amazing piece of behaviour in a troupe of Japanese macaque monkeys. Tourists threw pieces of sweet potato from a boat onto a local beach to attract the macaques. The macaques collected the food and tried to brush the sand off. Then one young female started to wash her pieces of sweet potato in the sea to remove the gritty sand. The behaviour quickly spread throughout the whole group. Only the adult males didn't copy this behaviour, although the young males soon followed their mothers and sisters!

Behaviour on the move

Some of the most dramatic animal behaviour is the mass migration of birds and mammals over thousands of kilometres. They travel in response to changes in the external environment, such as day length or temperature, or the need to reproduce. The migrations are almost completely instinctive. Some birds, such as geese, migrate for the first time in a family group, and seem to learn the route. In other species, such as cuckoos, the young birds migrate independently right from the start.

Many animal behaviours involve temperature regulation. Insects and reptiles cannot control their own temperature using heat from the reactions in the body. They orientate themselves to make the most of the warmth of the early morning sun to heat themselves up and get moving. Later, as the temperature gets hotter and hotter, they move into the shade to avoid overheating.

Penguins can control their own body temperature internally but live in such extreme conditions that they need to cluster together to conserve heat. These huddled chicks stand a much better chance of survival than if they stood alone.

Studying behaviour

Investigating animal behaviour

Everyone knows something about how animals and humans behave because it is part of our everyday lives. To really understand behaviour, scientists need to do more than watch their pet cat or observe their neighbours walking down the road.

Finding out how animals behave

Scientists have studied many different types of animal behaviour, from courtship and mating to memory and learning. American psychologist Burrhus Frederic Skinner played a very important part in investigating animal behaviour. He studied the way animals learn, and invented the Skinner box. This box can be used to hold an animal such as a pigeon or a rat. There is a button for the animal to press, a tray for it to

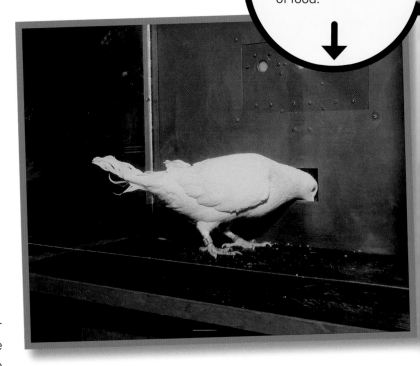

A pigeon in a Skinner box soon learns what to do to get a reward of food.

receive a reward of food or water, and a way for the scientist to change the conditions. Skinner showed that animals learnt new behaviours very quickly when they were rewarded. For example, pigeons could be taught to choose between a bright and a dim spot of light to get their reward.

Animals such as rats and pigeons are still used to study behaviour in a laboratory. They are cheap and easy to look after. Most people do not object to scientists working with these small animals if they are treated in a humane way. However, animals in laboratory conditions may not behave in the same way as they would do naturally. Therefore, observations of animals in the wild are very important.

Jane Goodall and the chimpanzees of Gombe

Chimpanzees are more like humans than any other animals. British **ethologist** Jane Goodall was one of the first people to carry out detailed research into chimpanzee family and social life. In the 1960s, she set up a long-term study of a group of chimpanzees at Gombe in Tanzania, Africa. She also helped American zoologist Dian Fossey who set up a similar research project into the behaviour of mountain gorillas. German Professor Biruté Galdikas also worked with the great apes, studying orangutans. Observing apes in the wild gives scientists a way of **evaluating** the information they collect from animals in zoos and in laboratories.

A chimpanzee uses a stick to fish for termites. Jane Goodall was the first person to report tool-making and tool-using in chimpanzees. Until then, everyone thought that only humans made tools.

THE SCIENCE YOU LEARN:
SCIENTIFIC INVESTIGATION

In science lessons you learn how to form a hypothesis and test it using experiments. You must keep conditions the same and only change the factor you are investigating. You need to think about the accuracy and reliability of your evidence. Are your results similar to others in the class, or are they very different? Is this because you are the only one who has got it right, or is there a mistake in your method? Scientists studying behaviour have to consider the same sort of problems. However, it is not easy to set up and control experiments on behaviour, especially when they involve humans.

Investigating human behaviour

To really understand human behaviour, scientists need to observe them carefully. For example, newborn babies behave in similar ways all over the world. They sleep, stretch, cry, and soon start to smile. They have reflexes – they blink and they grip tightly to anything placed in their hands.

In the same way, certain patterns of behaviour are recognizable in all adults. However, there are far more differences in the way adult humans behave. This is true not just in different countries and communities, but even within the same family.

Internal factors

There are more than 6 billion people on Earth. Apart from identical twins, each one has a different set of genetic instructions. Although everyone is different, we all have a lot of genetic information in common. Some of that genetic information influences our behaviour.

Humans have a number of behaviour patterns that are inherited. These are called **innate** or instinctive behaviours. A lot of human behaviour is built up as we learn from the responses to our innate behaviour.

Some of the most basic aspects of human behaviour are programmed into our genes and can be seen in very young babies.

For example, many facial expressions start off as innate. A newborn baby does not smile. Within a short time, a smile appears as an innate response to a pleasurable sensation such as being cuddled by its parents. This smile immediately gets a very positive response from the parent. This reinforces the innate behaviour, and the baby soon learns that a smile is a good way to get lots of attention.

Personality also seems to have a strong genetic link. **Longitudinal studies** (a series of observations carried out on the same people over many years) have shown that some strong personality traits can be seen in very young children. Some children are easy-going and happy, others are more likely to cry and be sad. As the children grow, these basic personality types remain, although they may change depending on what happens to the children as they grow. In fact at least 50 percent of the way you behave is probably down to your genes. The rest is the result of external factors – and this is what makes us all so different.

THE SCIENCE YOU LEARN: INHERITANCE AND GENETICS

DNA (genetic material) is found inside the nucleus in each cell of your body. The DNA is arranged into long strands called **chromosomes**. Along these chromosomes are the **genes**. The genes control the inheritance (passing on) of different features. Half of the genetic information is inherited from the mother, and half from the father. Genes have a strong influence on physical appearance such as eye colour and hair colour. In recent years scientists have found that some human behaviour may also have strong genetic links.

External factors and human behaviour

Within each country, and within each family, the external factors that affect human behaviour differ. Even identical twins have different positions in the family and are treated slightly differently. What sort of external factors affect human behaviour?

Bringing up baby

There is a lot of research that suggests that the way children are brought up affects their behaviour throughout the rest of their lives. Most children are lucky enough to have parents who try their best as they raise their family. The idea of what is best varies between **cultures**, but if children feel valued and loved they will respond. Children need contact with other humans. Parents, siblings, grandparents, friends, and other carers, and the chance to try new experiences, all help children to develop healthy behaviour patterns.

A child who is regularly beaten, or who sees other people hurt, is more likely to treat others badly. However, many children from harsh backgrounds make a great success of their lives and relationships. Children from "good" homes can behave in very destructive ways, turning to crime and drugs. So what else influences human behaviour?

CUTTING EDGE: RESISTING PEER PRESSURE

Recent research at Nottingham University has shown that some teenagers have an advantage when it comes to resisting peer pressure. Many teenagers were shown pictures of angry young people. The teenagers' brains showed lots of activity in the areas linked to getting information from the environment. In some of the teenagers there was also a lot of activity in the area involved in decision making. These teenagers were less likely to be influenced by their friends.

From a very early age, children want to behave in the same way as their peer group. The approval of friends is very important.

Peer pressure

The influence of peers (group of people of a similar age with whom you spend a lot of time) has a big effect on the way humans behave. From an early age, children form like-minded groups. It can be very hard if a child does not fit in. Children are very quick to be unkind to others who are different. The importance of a peer group cannot be underestimated. If parents value education and want a child to succeed, but the child has a group of friends who think it is stupid to work hard at school, it is likely that the child's school work will suffer. The child is not likely to give up the friends.

Peer pressure can be a great influence for good, or it can carry young people (and adults) into crime, alcohol, and drugs.

The environment also influences behaviour. For example, it is not possible to spend hours in front of a television if you have to walk several kilometres every day to collect water. It is not easy to decide exactly what affects human behaviour – there are lots of factors to take into account.

Nature versus nurture?

For many years, scientists have debated whether the way people behave is mainly the result of nature (their biology) or whether it is the result of nurture (the way they are brought up). At the moment, the evidence suggests that both are important.

It is possible to find out how a change in the environment, such as not enough food, a loud noise, or overcrowding, affects behaviour, by setting up an experiment. Or an investigation can be set up to see whether reward or punishment encourages faster learning. However, care needs to be taken as experiments need to be ethical, with no harm to animals.

It would be completely unethical to deprive babies of love to see if they behave differently. No-one would be allowed to make humans live in very overcrowded conditions to see if they became more aggressive. It would be interesting to see if some humans have a genetic makeup that means they are more likely to become addicted to alcohol. However it would be completely unacceptable to make a group of people drink large amounts of alcohol every day to see how many of them became addicted!

Overcoming the problems – twin studies

One way to overcome the problems of investigating human behaviour is to look at evidence from large numbers of people. If this is combined with taking observations over a period of years, the results can be very reliable.

Identical twins are particularly useful for studying behaviour because any differences in the way they behave must be down to nurture. Identical twins who have been separated from birth are most useful of all. Although this is relatively unusual, there are quite a few cases where it has happened.

When these twins are reunited, scientists can measure the similarities and differences between them. This gives a real insight into which aspects of their behaviour are inherited and which are the result of the way they have been brought up.

The data below is based on a groundbreaking study carried out at the University of Chicago, USA, in 1937. The researchers looked at 50 pairs of identical twins reared together, 50 pairs of identical twins reared apart, 50 pairs of non-identical twins, and 50 pairs of non-twin siblings. Some features, such as height, seem to be strongly genetic. Other features, such as mass, seem to be affected by nurture and behaviour – for example, how much you eat. Intelligence seems to be a mixture – both inherited and then affected by upbringing and opportunities.

Trait	Identical twins reared together	Identical twins reared apart	Non-identical twins	Non-twin siblings
Height difference	1.7 cm (0.6 in)	1.8 cm (0.7 in)	4.4 cm (1.7 in)	4.5 cm (1.8 in)
Mass difference	1.9 kg (4.2 lbs)	4.5 kg (9.9 lbs)	4.6 kg (10.1 lbs)	4.7 kg (10.4 lbs)
IQ score difference	5.9	8.2	9.9	9.8

THE SCIENCE YOU LEARN: IDENTICAL TWINS

At the moment of conception, a sperm fertilizes an egg. The new cell or zygote starts to divide to form a baby. Sometimes, during the first few divisions, the ball of cells that forms the early embryo splits completely in two. Both groups of cells continue to grow and form two embryos with identical genetic information. The embryos continue to grow and develop to form genetically identical babies.

Identical genetic information means that identical twins look very similar indeed.

The changing study of behaviour

The way behaviour is studied has changed over time. Many years ago it would have been unthinkable to consider animal behaviour and human behaviour together. Now it is recognized that we can learn a lot about how humans behave by looking at animals.

In the past, it was believed that you could tell whether someone was a criminal by measuring the lumps and bumps on their head! Now we understand that both genetics and the environment have an effect on behaviour (see pages 18-19).

As understanding grows about the causes of many diseases, our knowledge of the links between behaviour and health has also improved. It is well-known that smoking cigarettes is linked to an increased risk of lung cancer and heart disease. In the same way, food choices affect health as high fat, high calorie diets seem to be linked to obesity and heart disease.

Neuroscience, psychology, and psychiatry

The study of human behaviour falls into several different groups:

Neuroscientists study the nervous system. They look at the structure, development, and function of the nervous system. They observe how diseases affect the brain. Studying the brain and the rest of the nervous system involves studying how humans behave. Activity in the nervous system usually shows up as behaviour.

Psychology is the study of the mind. It is not possible to see what is going on in the mind, so psychologists rely on studying the way people behave. This gives them insights into the way the mind works.

Psychiatry is a branch of medicine. Psychiatrists study mental disorders in humans. They try to treat and, if possible, prevent mental health problems. They look at how human behaviour changes when the balance of the mind is altered, and try to find ways to help people maintain healthy minds and behaviours.

Normal behaviour and infant care

In the 1950s and 60s, American psychologist Harry Harlow carried out work on baby monkeys. At the time, it was thought that children bonded to their mothers because their mothers fed them. Baby rhesus monkeys were taken from their mothers and put in cages. In each cage were two fake mothers. One was made of wire and provided a bottle of milk. The other had no milk, but was covered in warm, cuddly material. The babies spent as little time as possible on the wire mother, only visiting her to feed. They spent most of their time on the cuddly mother. Harlow suggested that cuddling and contact were very important for normal development. The work Harry Harlow carried out on rhesus monkeys showed that interactions with lots of different animals was important for normal behaviour to develop. This also enhanced our knowledge of how human parents and babies interact.

Harry Harlow's experiments demonstrated that young monkeys need their real mothers if they are to develop and behave normally. They also need other monkeys to play and interact with.

Territory, ownership, and personal space

Aggression and display

Animals need space. They need places to raise their young, space to feed, and space to attract a mate. This space is known as their **territory**. Both territory and mates can be in short supply. Many animals show aggressive behaviour when they try to gain territory or a mate, and hold on to them. Food can also be a trigger for aggression. Some animals either attack another animal to kill it or to steal its food. Animals can also be agressive when they defend their food.

Aggression in animals

Aggression is behaviour that intimidates, frightens, or hurts another animal. Your pet dog may growl or bark when someone comes to the door. This is threatening behaviour, aggression designed to defend the territory. If an animal is badly frightened it may become aggressive as a form of defence.

In a herd of wild horses or ponies, the stallions (male horses) show aggression and fight each other over ownership of the mares (female horses). The mares can also be aggressive. There is a strict social order and the **dominant** mares may kick out at lower-ranking horses who do not show enough respect.

Stags fight during the rut (mating season) as they compete for territory and females. This aggression can lead to serious injury and even death.

Reducing the risk

Fighting carries the risk of injury and death. Therefore, many species of animals have developed a less dangerous form of aggressive behaviour. Behavioural displays are used to make a point instead of the use of physical violence.

There are many examples of behaviour that allow animals to avoid aggression. Marking territory warns other animals that a patch of land is already claimed. Territory marking comes in many forms. It can involve using scent from special glands, urine, or faeces. When a pet cat rubs her head against her owner she is marking the owner as "hers". In the same way, a male tiger sprays urine against a tree to tell other male tigers to keep away from his land. Territory marking can also involve sound. Birdsong can be a way of telling other birds to keep away from a particular territory.

Some animals, such as wildebeest and buffalo, form large social herds. Other animals, such as chimpanzees and gorillas, form smaller groups. In these groups, there is often a **hierarchy**. The animals at the top have got there by very aggressive behaviour. However, it would be exhausting and dangerous to be aggressive all the time, and instead very complex social signals have developed. These signals allow the dominant animals to use displays to show that they are at the top. It also means lower-ranking animals can show they accept being less important by displaying to the dominant animals. This means the damage done to individuals is kept to a minimum.

These are some of the signals that animals use to avoid outright aggression.

Human aggression and crime

Aggression in humans includes fighting, road rage, domestic violence, muggings, murder, and war. Many of the triggers for aggressive behaviour are similar in humans and animals. In theory, humans are intelligent and can think things through, so there should be less aggression in human society than in animal groups. In fact, aggression is surprisingly common.

Aggressive behaviour over territory, belongings, and food is seen in very young children. Adults can have disputes over boundaries that last years. Wars are fought over territory. The territory can be land, or oil, or ideas – but aggression on the level of whole armies is very frightening.

Just like animals, humans have developed many rituals and displays that can be used instead of physical violence. Language means that people can be very aggressive without lifting a finger.

We use signals such as possessions and lifestyle to make statements about ourselves. Body language also sends out signals. Smiling, holding doors open, and thousands of other examples of behaviour can be used to indicate how dominant we are feeling. Humans avoid aggression by either acknowledging another human's place in the pecking order (social status) or by asserting their own in a non-threatening way.

Crime is often linked with aggression. Why some people become aggressive and/or criminal is not fully understood. Scientists are gathering more and more evidence that both our genetics and our environment affect how aggressive we become.

This graph shows you the trends in recorded violent crime in several countries per 100,000 people between 1962 and 2004. When you remember that the total population of each of these countries runs into millions, you can see that hundreds of thousands of people are the victims of aggressive criminal human behaviour every year.

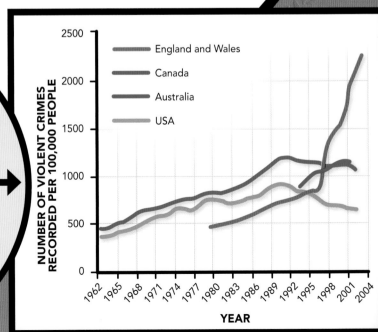

Nature, nurture, and criminal behaviour

In the early 21st century, scientists published the results of a study on around 1,000 children in New Zealand, taken over a period of 23 years. They were looking for links between genes and upbringing. They measured many things, including the levels of a chemical called **monoamine oxidase (MAOA)**. MAOA breaks down chemical messengers in the brain. High levels of MAOA seem to be linked to depression. Low MAOA levels seem to be linked to aggressive behaviour. The level of MAOA someone makes is inherited.

No one has to be a criminal and end up in a prison like this one. However, evidence suggests that the genes we inherit may make some of us more likely to be aggressive and violent than others, and so more likely to commit a crime.

The scientists found a clear **correlation** between the way children coped with being treated badly and their MAOA levels. Those who suffered bad treatment as children but had high MAOA levels were no more likely to be violent or criminal than anyone else. However, those who had low MAOA and were badly treated seemed to be worse affected. They only made up 12 percent of the group, but they made up 44 percent of the people convicted of violent crime.

The gene for MAOA is inherited on the chromosomes that determine gender, and problems are more common in men. This may help explain why males are more likely than females to be involved in aggressive and criminal behaviour. The evidence from this study suggests that an interaction between genes (the level of MAOA in the brain) and environment (whether or not someone is badly treated as a child) may affect how aggressive they are as an adult.

Human behaviour throughout life

The early years

When human babies are born they are completely dependent on adults to look after them. Without this care, the baby will die. The behaviour of babies is largely the result of reflex responses and instincts. Some of the behaviours are simple reflexes. The rooting response is a simple reflex. The baby turns its head and open its mouth to search for food. Other simple patterns of behaviour encourage parents to respond to and look after their baby. They are known as signalling behaviours because they send clear signals to the carers. When a baby is hungry, cold, or unhappy, it will cry. When someone comforts or feeds the baby, the crying stops. Clear evidence suggests that when carers respond quickly to a crying baby, the baby cries less. It soon learns to trust that help will come when it is needed.

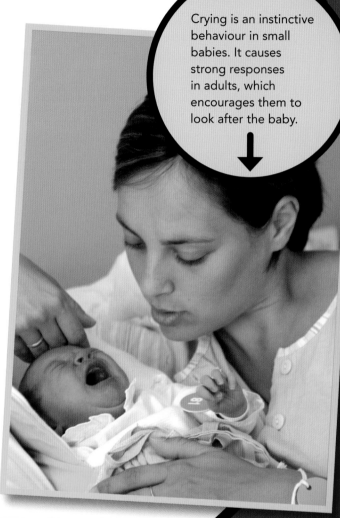

Crying is an instinctive behaviour in small babies. It causes strong responses in adults, which encourages them to look after the baby.

CUTTING EDGE: THE PHYSICAL RESPONSE TO CRYING

The sound of a baby crying has a physical effect on adults, whether they are parents or not. American scientist Ann Frodi at the University of Rochester, USA, has carried out tests on the effect of crying on parents, childless adults, teenagers, and even children as young as eight years old.

When they heard a baby crying, they all showed an increase in heart rate and blood pressure and a change in the way their skin conducts electricity. Everyone described anxiety and irritation at the sound, and a desire to make it stop.

How does behaviour develop?

The way children learn to behave depends on a number of things. Teaching and learning is very important. Parents, grandparents, other carers, teachers at school, and even older brothers and sisters all teach a child how to behave. These lessons vary from simply learning the skills needed to look after yourself – bowel and bladder control, teeth cleaning, and how to put on shoes – through to manners, cooperation, and self-control.

One important way in which children learn is through observation and copying. It is not just simple behaviours that are copied. Children learn morals from their parents from a very early age. For example, children from a considerate home are likely to be thoughtful of others, whereas children who see violence are more likely to hit out to solve their own problems.

Mimicry (copying) plays a big part in the way children learn to behave.

Toddlers and children

As babies grow into toddlers, and toddlers grow into children, behaviour changes from instincts and reflexes to much more learned and conscious behaviour. The development of social skills is an important area of behaviour. If a child learns to interact happily with its carers, other adults, and other children, the basis for mental and physical health and stability is laid.

Adolescence to adulthood

The behaviour of children affects their health. Children are naturally inquisitive and active, busy playing and exploring their environment. However, more and more children in the United Kingdom and United States spend a lot of time watching television and playing computer games. The food they eat is often high in fats and sugars. As a result, increasing numbers of children are becoming overweight or obese. This has a direct effect on their health. They get breathless, and are more likely to suffer from asthma and diabetes. In the future they may be more likely to develop heart disease and some cancers.

THE SCIENCE YOU LEARN: CHANGES AT PUBERTY

At puberty, the brain and sex organs (ovaries in girls, testes in boys) start to make chemical messages known as sex hormones. These hormones trigger all the other physical changes that occur at puberty such as growth, change in body shape, the start of periods (menstruation) in girls, and the production of sperm in boys.

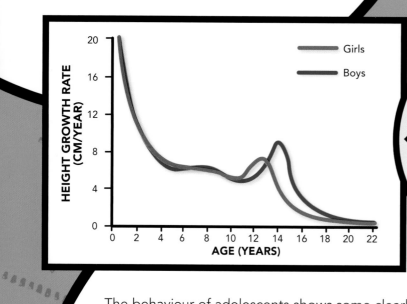

Your growth rate is fastest when you are a baby. It slows down a lot by the time you are about three years old. During puberty your growth rate increases as you grow from being a child to an adult.

The behaviour of adolescents shows some clearly defined patterns. Teenagers find it harder to get to sleep. Therefore they go to bed later, but as they are growing fast they need lots of sleep. As a result, they tend to wake up late and groggy in the mornings. Peer-group relationships become more and more important as teenagers distance themselves from family ties. They become more independent. At this point real dangers can appear. Binge drinking, drug taking, and violent behaviour are increasingly seen in teenagers, and often peer pressure is part of the problem. Behaviour like this can have serious health consequences in both the short and the long term (see pages 44-47).

Teenagers can also have problems with empathy, which means they find it difficult to understand the points of view of other people. Yet they can also be caring, compassionate, and idealistic. While a teenager can experience powerful mood swings as a result of the brain restructuring that is going on, they find it more difficult to recognize emotions in other people.

Sexual behaviour is an important part of adolescent development. The sexes become much more aware of each other. Finding a boyfriend or girlfriend and sexual behaviour take up increasing amounts of time and thought.

In a teenager's brain, many different nerve connections are being removed or reformed. In particular, changes take place in parts of the brain concerned with emotion and motivation. The teenage brain can have real problems in assessing risks. The risky, daredevil behaviour of some young people is often seen as rebellion or wildness. It may simply be an inability to make the connection between behaviour such as driving recklessly or drug taking, and the possible consequences.

"The thing that is really irritating about teenagers ... is that one moment their behaviour is that of adults, while the next it is that of a not very bright three-year-old ... or an amoeba! The rapid oscillation [change] between child and adult is one of the hallmarks of the teenager." [Vivienne Parry, British scientist, journalist, and broadcaster.]

Adulthood and old age

Human adult behaviour is very varied. This is partly because adult behaviour depends strongly on the culture to which a person belongs. The behaviour of adult women in an American city will be very different from the behaviour of adult women in a remote Indian village, for example. Masai warriors in Africa will behave very differently to British farmers. Many of these differences are examples of learned behaviour. A child born in one community, but raised in the traditions of another, will show the behaviour patterns of the place where they grew up.

Some types of behaviour are common to adults in almost every culture. Sexual behaviour is one (see pages 32–37). Parenting behaviour is another. The details of parenting behaviour vary between cultures, but there are some common threads. Mothers usually nurture their children. They either breastfeed their infants or bottle-feed artificial milk formula. In many cultures women do most of the child rearing, so much of the behaviour learnt by very young children comes from their mothers. The role of fathers in raising children varies widely across cultures. A very involved approach is encouraged in the United Kingdom and the United States at the moment, but in other communities men take little or no part in child rearing.

Adults usually work, either for money or to maintain a home and feed a family. Adult behaviour also involves self-control, the ability to empathize with others, and the ability to plan and take charge. In adult communities, some people are more dominant than others. This can be seen clearly in the workplace and in the home.

The choices adults make about their behaviour in everyday life – the food they eat, what they drink, the exercise they take, and whether they smoke or use drugs – all have a big effect on their health and well-being (see pages 42–47).

Ageing

As humans age, physical changes can affect the way they behave. Muscles weaken, eyesight and hearing worsen, healing takes longer, and memory may begin to fail. All of these things can reduce a person's confidence, and affect the way they behave. People may be just as capable of enjoying a game of football when they are 70 years old as when they were 40, or even 20. But the fear of injury, or of not seeing the ball clearly, often means that older people withdraw from sports and other activities. Yet maintaining normal active behaviour is one of the most important ways of staying healthy into old age. It keeps the muscles as strong as possible, and reduces the chance of heart disease. Keeping active also helps people keep their weight down and makes them less likely to have diseases such as diabetes and arthritis. Enjoying life and keeping mentally active helps to reduce the likelihood of memory loss or depression.

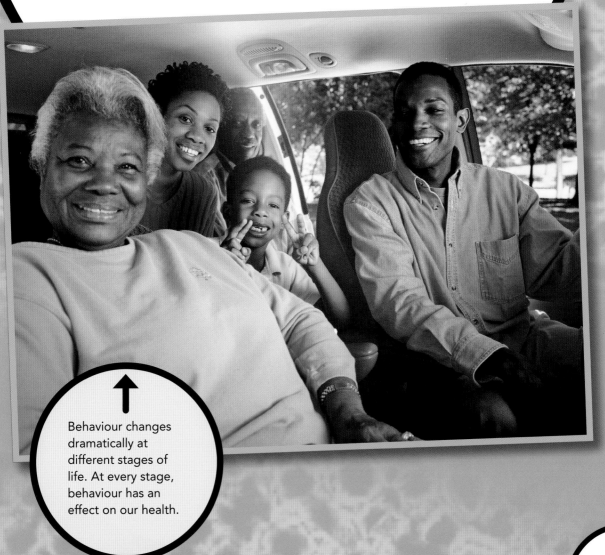

Behaviour changes dramatically at different stages of life. At every stage, behaviour has an effect on our health.

Sexual behaviour

Courtship and mating in the animal world

Many animals do not mate. Instead they release their sex cells into water. Animals that live on land have to mate to pass the male sex cells into the female body to meet the egg. In many animals, finding a partner and mating involves some very complex behaviour. Most of this behaviour is instinctive or innate rather than learned, although most animals get better at it with practice.

Courtship displays

Male and female animals, including humans, are often looking for different things when it comes to reproduction. Males make huge quantities of very small sex cells. They want to mate with many females and father as many offspring as possible. Females make a limited number of much larger sex (egg) cells. It takes a lot of resources to make eggs and a big time investment in the developing young. Therefore, females look for a small number of partners, but they are looking for the best possible mates. They need the best genetic material so their offspring have a good chance of survival. A mate with a large territory means there will be lots of food for the offspring. A mate who will help to rear the young means the offspring are more likely to survive.

Many animals have courtship rituals, where the males display in some way and the females choose their mates. Courtship displays may rely on sight and/or sound. Many also depend on scent. Chemicals called **pheromones** are produced and these attract the opposite sex. Unlike humans, most female animals are only prepared to mate when they are fertile, so male animals also rely on scent to tell them when a female is ready to mate.

The dangers of mating

Once courtship is over and a mate is chosen, the animals will mate. This can be very dangerous. For many female animals it means allowing another potentially dangerous animal to come extremely close to you. She will be within easy reach of claws, jaws, and teeth. For this reason, during mating, some animals like to make sure that their partner is occupied and already has something to eat. Praying mantises and a number of spiders famously eat their mates during the act of mating unless they are successfully distracted.

Animal courtship rituals

In some species of hangingflies, the males offer the females a dead insect to eat while mating. This proves they are good providers. The bigger the dead insect, the longer the female will mate, and the more eggs the male can fertilize.

Male birds of paradise have beautiful feathers and often have complicated mating dances. They use the dances to display their feathers to attract a female.

The fights between male elephant seals for territory and females can leave both animals injured and many seal pups are crushed during the battle.

The display of a male bird of paradise is designed to convince a female that he would be a good father for her offspring.

Human sexual behaviour

Just like other animals, human sexual behaviour is all about attracting a mate. Unlike many other animals, humans can choose to be sexually active at any point during the menstrual cycle.

Sexual behaviour is not simple. It is a mixture of innate patterns caused by hormones inside the body, responses to signals from other humans, and learnt behaviour. Humans learn about sexual behaviour by watching others, from characters in films to their parents.

Human displays

In many ways, human courtship is very different from animals because we use the higher centres of our brain and think carefully about what we are doing. Humans live as part of a society, and a mate who is well regarded in society is very valuable. In many human societies, sex is closely linked to marriage, when a man and a woman form a partnership. However, when it comes to sex, in some ways we are still very much like animals and respond strongly to certain signals.

Some of the signals that humans respond to are obvious. Appearance is very important in human sexual behaviour. This is why humans dress up for a night out! The way humans speak and the things they say are also important. Scent is another important aspect of human sexual behaviour, which is why perfume, deodorant, and aftershave sell so well. There are also other more subtle scents that our bodies respond to. Humans produce pheromones and detect these cues. In one piece of research, scientists sprayed male pheromones on certain chairs in a waiting room. Later, women only sat on the sprayed chairs. When the situation was reversed and female pheromones were used, men actively chose to sit on the sprayed chairs. Without any awareness of what was going on, people chose the chairs that gave out a message about sex!

The power of advertising

The sex drive in humans is very strong. In men, the sight of an attractive woman can very rapidly arouse desire. In women, the situation is more complex, although physical appearance is important. The advertising and marketing industries use these responses because using sex in adverts sells products. This is partly because the images make people take notice of the advert. The images also suggest that if you use a certain product, you too will be sexually successful. In advertising directed at men, beautiful women are often involved. The subtle message is: Buy this product and you will attract beautiful women. In advertising that targets women, good-looking men and romance often feature. The biological message that works for women is: Buy this product and you will attract good-looking, rich, successful men who will father healthy children and help you take care of them!

Sexual behaviour in humans, from a Valentine's day dinner to an expensive wedding, is part of a huge industry. Yet in biological terms, sexual behaviour is still all about selecting a mate and producing healthy babies.

Sexual health

Humans do not have sexual intercourse only to conceive offspring. In fact, many do not want to risk getting pregnant every time they have sex. One important form of human sexual behaviour is the use of **contraception**. Contraception literally means against conception. Barrier methods of contraception, such as the condom, stop the sperm from reaching the egg. The pill is a chemical method of contraception.

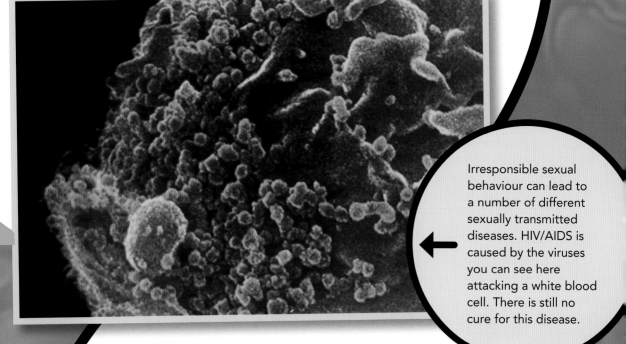

Irresponsible sexual behaviour can lead to a number of different sexually transmitted diseases. HIV/AIDS is caused by the viruses you can see here attacking a white blood cell. There is still no cure for this disease.

Sexually transmitted diseases

One result of human sexual behaviour is the spread of **sexually transmitted diseases (STDs)**. An STD is passed from one person to another through sex. Anyone who is sexually active can catch an STD.

In their early stages, they most commonly affect the sex organs. In many cases, untreated STDs can cause **infertility**. Some, like syphilis, can cause serious illness and death. The human papilloma virus causes genital warts. These affect men and women and are unpleasant but not usually serious. However, the same virus has been shown to cause cervical cancer in women. This cancer can be treated successfully if it is discovered early, but thousands of women still die from it every year. A vaccine is now available, which is given to young people before they become sexually active to protect them from the virus.

Perhaps the best-known result of dangerous sexual behaviour is HIV/AIDS, a viral disease that attacks the body's defence system. So far, although new medicines can help people live much longer, there is no cure or vaccine for this disease.

Most STDs can be treated, and if they are caught early they have no long-term effects. Unfortunately it is not easy to tell if someone has an STD. Many STDs do not cause major symptoms for years, and if someone catches one it is easy to miss the early symptoms. Humans can carry an STD for years, passing it on to their sexual partners until they become seriously ill or realize they are infertile. Sensible sexual behaviour is vital to avoid the problems of STDs. That includes having only one sexual partner and using barrier contraception with a new partner. Ideally barrier methods should be used until both partners have had tests to show that they are free from STDs.

SCIENCE YOU LEARN: CONCEPTION TO BIRTH

During sexual intercourse, the male sperm (sex cells) are released inside the body of the female. They move through the uterus into the Fallopian tubes. If an egg (the female sex cell) has been released from the ovary, the sperm will cluster around the egg. Eventually one sperm may penetrate the protective coat of the egg. This is the moment of conception, when a potential new life begins. The fertilized egg begins to divide and over nine months becomes a fully developed baby.

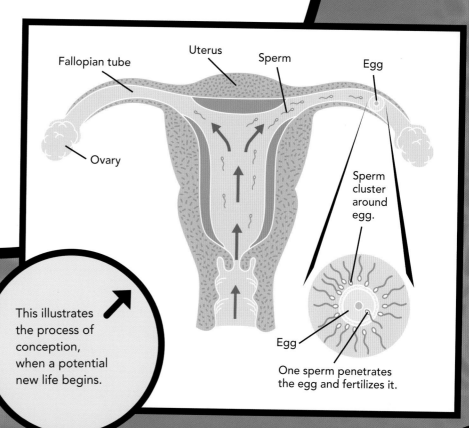

Fallopian tube

Uterus

Sperm

Egg

Ovary

Sperm cluster around egg.

Egg

One sperm penetrates the egg and fertilizes it.

This illustrates the process of conception, when a potential new life begins.

Health and behaviour

Eating too much – or too little

In countries such as the United States, the United Kingdom, and Australia there is plenty of food, much of it cheap and often high in calories. Many people eat a healthy, balanced diet but eating behaviour is changing. The modern trend is to graze throughout the day on high-energy snacks, coffee, and fast food. As a result, people are getting fatter. There is good scientific evidence that increasing weight is linked to health problems such as heart disease and diabetes.

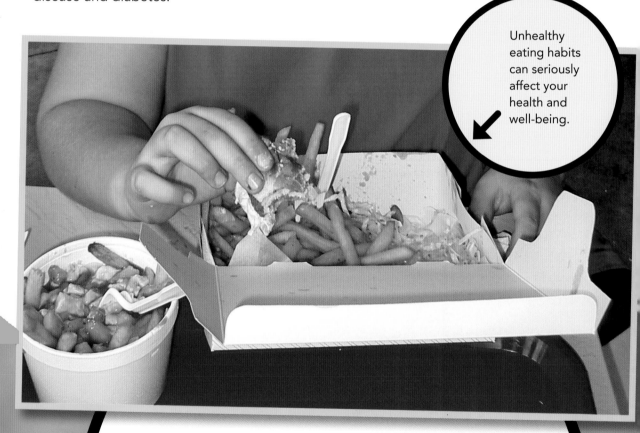

Unhealthy eating habits can seriously affect your health and well-being.

Some people eat too much, but others eat too little. Eating behaviour becomes distorted when people deliberately starve themselves. This eating disorder is called anorexia nervosa. Eating disorders are mental illnesses in which people perceive themselves as fat even when they are dangerously thin. They feel they need to control everything that goes into and out of the body.

Does food affect health?

There is increasing evidence that a diet high in fruit and vegetables can help protect you against heart disease and a number of different cancers. A diet that is high in animal fats, such as butter and cream, seems to be linked to an increased risk of heart disease and cancers. The amount of salt in your diet can affect your blood pressure, although only some people are sensitive to salt levels. There is still a lot to discover about the links between eating behaviour and health. How do scientists find out what is going on?

INVESTIGATION PANEL:
LOOKING FOR CAUSE AND EFFECT

Finding out how human behaviour affects health is not easy. You cannot easily experiment on humans. To show that a particular behaviour causes certain health effects, scientists need to look at data (information) from thousands of people. For example, The National Children's Study has been set up in the United States. The aim is to investigate genetic influences and environmental influences, such as diet, social setting, and education, on children's health and well-being. Much of the funding is coming from the United States government.

More than 100,000 children will be observed in 105 different study centres. The children will come from right across the United States so that every different ethnic group is included. The children will be observed from before birth (when their mothers are pregnant) until they are 21 years old.

Scientists will collect the information through interviews with the mothers, and with the children as they get older. They will also use questionnaires and examine the health and development of the children at regular intervals. At the end of the study, scientists hope to identify which factors in the behaviour of pregnant women and in the way children are fed and brought up help to make them healthier for the rest of their lives.

Similar studies have been carried out and are happening in many other countries.

Stress, exercise, and health

Modern life is very busy. In school there is constant pressure to achieve and fit in. For adults there are the demands of work, home, family, and friends. Most of the time, these stresses are a good thing. They give a sense of purpose, excitement, and challenge. However, sometimes the pressure is too much, or goes on for too long. Then it can lead to illness, with both physical and emotional problems. Millions of people visit their doctor each year with stress-related problems.

For severe problems a doctor will prescribe medicine, but many people manage to overcome their stress without drugs. They may go on holiday, or take up a relaxing hobby. Lots of people take up exercise, from yoga to running. Exercise relieves stress. It is physically demanding and takes your mind off the stress. It is tiring, which is why it helps people to sleep. Exercise also triggers the release of feel-good chemicals in the brain known as endorphins, which can cause feelings of happiness.

Exercise is good for both your mental and physical health. →

Exercise and health

Exercise is also important for good health in many other ways. Lots of people take very little exercise. They may prefer to watch television or use the computer. Yet scientific evidence shows that people who take regular exercise are healthier. They are less likely to be affected by heart disease and a disease called osteoporosis in which the bones become easy to break.

INVESTIGATION PANEL: HOW MUCH EXERCISE DO YOU DO?

Investigate the exercise levels in your local community, whether in school or at home.

Procedure

1. Write a short questionnaire designed to find out how much exercise people do. Reassure people that the questionnaire will be anonymous. Choose your questions carefully. Just asking "Do you exercise?" will not tell you much. Useful questions include "How many times do you exercise for more than 20 minutes each week?" and "Do you walk or cycle to work?" Record the age and sex of the people who complete your questionnaire.

2. Decide how many questionnaires you are going to use. The more you fill in, the more reliable your results will be, but the more data you will have to deal with. Hand out your questionnaires.

3. Analyze the data you have collected. For example, you could produce a bar chart to show the number of times people exercise in a week. You could draw a pie chart to show the percentage of people who walk or cycle to work or school compared to those taking the bus, car, or train.

4. Look at your data and draw conclusions about the activity levels of the people you have studied. Are they active and healthy or do they need to take more exercise? If they need to take more, how could you persuade them to do so?

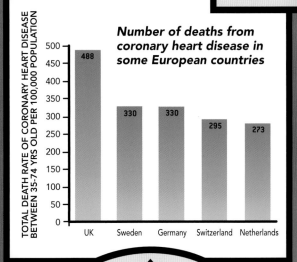

Graph A

Number of deaths from coronary heart disease in some European countries

TOTAL DEATH RATE OF CORONARY HEART DISEASE BETWEEN 35-74 YRS OLD PER 100,000 POPULATION

UK 488, Sweden 330, Germany 330, Switzerland 295, Netherlands 273

Graph A shows the number of deaths from heart disease in several European countries. Graph B shows the percentage of journeys made by bicycle in the same countries. This gives a good idea of the level of exercise people take. There seems to be a link between exercise and heart health, although one piece of evidence does not prove or disprove a theory.

Graph B

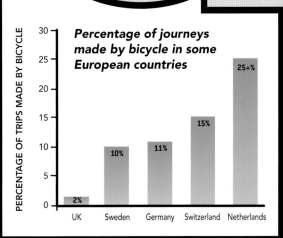

Percentage of journeys made by bicycle in some European countries

PERCENTAGE OF TRIPS MADE BY BICYCLE

UK 2%, Sweden 10%, Germany 11%, Switzerland 15%, Netherlands 25+%

Legal drugs, legal killers

A drug is a chemical that has a specific effect on your body. Many drugs are prescribed by doctors to help the body overcome diseases. Some, like painkillers and indigestion tablets, are sold at chemists.

Tea, coffee, cigarettes, and alcoholic drinks contain legal and commonly used drugs, but there are other drugs that are not legal to use. To make the right decisions about using legal and illegal drugs it is important to realize that both can damage health. In the United Kingdom, more than 100,000 people die from using alcohol each year, and another 100,000 die from smoking-related diseases.

Smoking is behaviour that has well-known bad effects on your health and appearance, yet millions of people continue to smoke.

Smoking

Around the world, millions of people smoke tobacco, most commonly as cigarettes. Cigarette smoke contains many different chemicals including a drug called nicotine. This drug stimulates the body but narrows the blood vessels. It makes people feel calmer and more able to cope with stress. However, the body becomes addicted to nicotine. As people get used to the drug, they need more nicotine to have the same effect, and therefore smoke more cigarettes.

Cigarette smoke also contains a thick black tar which builds up in the lungs. This tar makes smokers more likely to get bronchitis and other serious lung conditions. Smoking is also strongly linked to lung cancer. Up to 90 percent of all cases of lung cancer are caused by smoking. The heart is also affected by smoking, making a heart attack or stroke far more likely. Smoking ages the skin, and women who smoke when they are pregnant increase the risk of their baby dying.

Sir Richard Doll

Richard Doll was a British scientist who researched the link between smoking and lung cancer. He is famous for being the first person ever to provide a scientific link between the two. He worked at the United Kingdom Medical Research Council and published his groundbreaking paper in 1954. He gave up smoking himself during his study. Since then, thousands of studies have confirmed the links between smoking and many different health problems. Sir Richard Doll himself went on to study smoking-related diseases for more than 50 years.

Data like this has been collected over many years. The evidence against cigarettes is overwhelming.

Why smoke?

Most people begin smoking when they are fairly young. They may copy their parents, or start to smoke because it is regarded as cool, or rebellious. Yet other young people start to smoke as a result of pressure from their peer group – if your friends smoke, it can be hard to say no. Whatever the reasons for starting, the reason people continue to smoke is their addiction to nicotine. This is what makes it so hard to change smoking behaviour. It is far better not to start.

Alcohol – legal but dangerous

Alcohol is a social drug that is widely used in many parts of the world. When someone drinks an alcoholic drink, the alcohol passes into the bloodstream and into almost every tissue of the body, including the brain. It slows down thought processes and reflexes. All reactions become slower than normal.

A little alcohol can make people feel relaxed and at ease. It also leads to a lack of self control and a lack of judgement. More alcohol can cause aggression and a complete loss of control. The person may pass out and even die.

Alcohol is addictive. When people cannot cope without alcohol they are called alcoholics. Heavy alcohol use over a period of years can cause long-term damage to the brain. The brains of dead alcoholics are sometimes so soft and pulpy that almost all of the normal brain structures have been lost.

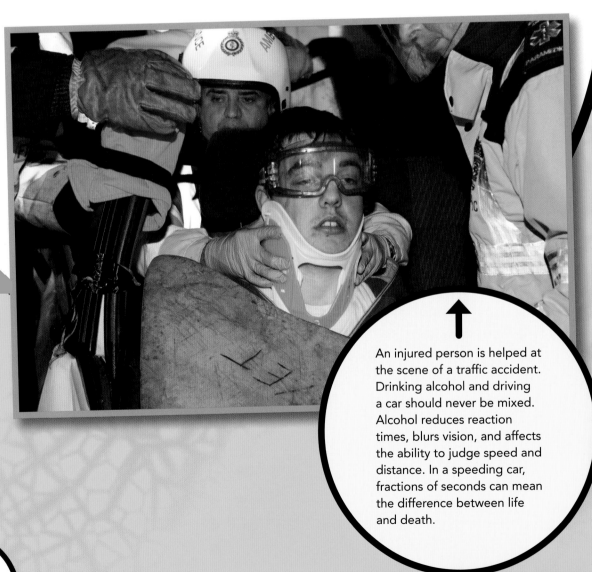

An injured person is helped at the scene of a traffic accident. Drinking alcohol and driving a car should never be mixed. Alcohol reduces reaction times, blurs vision, and affects the ability to judge speed and distance. In a speeding car, fractions of seconds can mean the difference between life and death.

Normally alcohol is broken down in the liver into harmless substances. People who drink very large amounts of alcohol, or who drink heavily for a long time, are at risk from potentially fatal liver diseases. These include cirrhosis of the liver and liver cancer.

Many non-drinkers also suffer from alcohol abuse. Drunken drivers kill people in road accidents. Violent crimes are committed after drinking. Families can break down as a result of one or both parents drinking heavily. If pregnant women drink too much alcohol, their baby may be born with disabilities.

People have drunk alcoholic drinks for centuries, but if the drug was discovered today it would probably be banned as too dangerous for use.

CASE STUDY

Binge drinking

Excessive alcohol consumption with the main purpose of getting drunk is called binge drinking. This has become a major problem in many countries of the world.

In the United Kingdom young people in particular often drink huge amounts of alcohol at weekends. This drinking is linked to antisocial behaviour, from loud, unpleasant scenes to serious violence. In 2005, a report in the United Kingdom showed that one million admissions to hospital accident and emergency units each year are alcohol linked.

In Australia there is a similar problem. There are cases where 13 and 14-year-olds have been involved in binge drinking. In older teenagers it is very common, even though the legal age for buying alcohol is 18.

In the United States the situation is slightly different. The national minimum drinking age is 21. Therefore binge drinking has become a sign of rebellion in teenagers and young adults. As it is illegal for them to drink, they have to break the law to get access to the alcohol in the first place.

All of these countries, and many others, are looking for ways to control this problem. They want to prevent the damage caused to individuals and society before it is too late.

Illegal drugs

Many illegal drugs have a powerful effect on the mind. Some produce hallucinations (like waking dreams), others give an overwhelming sense of happiness and power. Once people have experienced the drug's high, they want it again and again. Addicts may not be able to cope with life without the drug. It is very difficult to stop using drugs. If people give up the drug they feel extremely ill as they suffer from withdrawal symptoms.

Most illegal drugs can damage your health by causing heart failure and death. This can happen the first time you try a drug, or the 100th time. Illegal drugs are expensive. Addicts often get involved in crime to pay for their drugs. Many addicts damage their health because they live in great poverty. They spend all their money on drugs, rather than eating a balanced diet or keeping clean.

Spreading disease

Some drugs are injected straight into the bloodstream. Once addicts start injecting drugs they may share needles with other drug users. Serious diseases can be spread in this way. Blood infected with microbes can be passed from one person to another on dirty needles. Hepatitis, a serious disease of the liver, and HIV/AIDS are common amongst injecting drug addicts. In addition, if people are caught using or supplying illegal drugs they can be tried and sent to prison. In some parts of the world they are put to death.

So far, science has not found a way to overcome the cravings of a drug addict. There is relatively little money available to support research. The behaviour of an addict almost always damages their health, but the behaviour needed to overcome the addiction takes a lot of character and determination. Many people find this very hard.

Crystal meth

Crystal meth (methamphetamine) is a relatively new and inexpensive drug. It is snorted up the nose, injected, or smoked, and it acts as a stimulant. People feel high, very awake, alert, and happy for hours after using the drug. It also tends to make people very sexually active.

Crystal meth is also very destructive. It can have a very rapid damaging effect on both health and behaviour. It is psychologically very addictive, and it affects mental health and well-being. It can cause mood swings, paranoia, rage, and short-term memory loss. It damages the mouth and skin, leading to horrible sores. If people overdose on the drug, they can suffer a complete collapse of their circulatory and breathing systems, go into a coma, and die. People using crystal meth often also have a lot of sex with a lot of different people, putting them at risk of STDs. In the United States, for example, almost 50 percent of new cases of HIV/AIDS involve the use of crystal meth.

The use of crystal meth is spreading from the United States to the United Kingdom and many other countries.

These two photos of the same crystal meth addict were taken 18 months apart. The more recent photograph on the right clearly shows the woman's worsening physical condition.

Summary

Health and behaviour

Behaviour is the actions displayed by an organism in response to its environment. Behaviour is affected by factors inside and outside the body, and can be observed and measured. Animal behaviour involves everything that goes on in life, from eating and defending territories to raising young. It ranges from simple reflexes to complicated human actions such as developing the technology to send people into space.

In humans and many other larger animals, behaviour depends on three things. The senses provide information about the outside world and the inside of the body, the central nervous system analyzes the information, and nerves send messages out to the muscles, controlling movement.

The study of animal behaviour has taught us a great deal about the basis of human behaviour. Although much of human behaviour depends on conscious thought, a lot of instinct and innate behaviour is also involved in life. There are ethical problems with experimenting on humans, so a lot of work on human behaviour is carried out by large surveys. It is interesting to see how much of our behaviour is part of our genetic makeup, and how much is a result of the environment in which we grow up.

The way you behave and the choices you make directly affect your health. Choosing to eat lots of fat-rich food and avoid any exercise could mean that your arteries become narrow and even blocked.

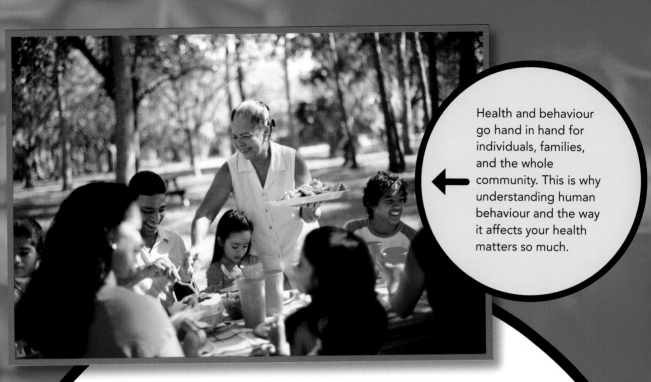

Health and behaviour go hand in hand for individuals, families, and the whole community. This is why understanding human behaviour and the way it affects your health matters so much.

There is no doubt that the way you behave affects your health. Your behaviour and responses change as you grow. A newborn baby is a mass of reflexes, but much adult behaviour is the result of conscious thought. Some human behaviour, such as aggressive tendencies, have their roots in animal behaviour. As people can think things through, these behaviours are often changed and used in different ways.

The food you choose to eat also has a major effect on your health. Too much food, too little, lots of fat, lots of fruit – all have effects on the health of your body.

Like all animals, one of the strongest drives in human behaviour is the desire to find a mate and produce offspring. Sexual behaviour also carries with it the risk of unwanted pregnancy and STDs.

Once people have children, parenting behaviour becomes very important if the baby is to grow up happy and secure. However it is not just upbringing that affects a child. As children grow up, the influence of their peer group becomes a big factor in the way they behave. Peer groups often influence whether people start smoking, drinking, or using illegal drugs. These chemicals affect the brain and alter behaviour. They can have devastating effects on health and well-being.

Many people don't know how much their behaviour affects their mental and physical health, but once you are aware, you can begin to make choices that will keep you as healthy as possible.

Leabharlanna Poibli Chathair Bhaile Átha Cliath

Facts and figures

Timeline of the study of behaviour

350 BC Greek philosopher Aristotle writes about memory and reminiscence as he tries to explain how people remember things.

1566 Bernardino Alvarez, a Spaniard who set up the Hospital do San Hipolito in Mexico, the first hospital in the Americas for patients with mental health problems.

1791 Italian scientist, Luigi Galvani, uses the muscles in frogs legs to show that nerve impulses are electrical.

1875 British scientist Francis Galton (Charles Darwin's cousin) introduces the use of twin studies in his book *History of Twins*.

1877 Charles Darwin, the great British scientist, publishes *Sketch of an Infant*, a detailed account of the development and behaviour of one of his own children.

1906 Russian scientist Ivan Pavlov publishes his famous experiments on conditioned reflexes in dogs.

1930s–50s Burrhus Skinner carries out his work on conditioning in rats and pigeons and many other aspects of behaviour.

1950s Konrad Lorenz (Austrian) and Nikolaas Tinbergen (Dutch) with Karl von Frisch (Austrian) develop the science of ethology, the study of animal behaviour in natural contexts.

1950s–60s American psychologist Harry Harlow carries out experiments on the mother-infant bond in rhesus monkeys.

1962–63 The first evidence is uncovered that physical changes in the brain take place when something is memorized.

1960s–70s Scientists Jane Goodall and Dian Fossey study the behaviour of chimpanzees and mountain gorillas, respectively.

1990s MRI scanning becomes available, allowing scientists to see what is happening inside the brain.

2002 Studies show how inherited levels of MAOA interact with the childhood environment to influence behaviour.

2007 Work in the United Kingdom and elsewhere suggests that some people resist peer pressure more easily than others.

Biographies

Burrhus Frederic Skinner

Born in 1904 in Pennsylvania, USA, Burrhus Frederic Skinner studied English literature before he became involved in animal behaviour. Burrhus had always enjoyed building things, and he quickly began to devise new apparatus for his investigations. It wasn't long before his famous Skinner box was produced (see page 12). By 1938 he had published his first book on behaviour. During World War II, Skinner worked on a top secret project, training pigeons to guide bombs.

In 1948 he joined the Psychology Department at Harvard University and stayed there for the rest of his working life. He also became involved in education after he discovered that the way children were taught maths went against everything he had discovered about the way animals learn. He spent many years developing improved ways of teaching children in schools. Skinner died of leukaemia in 1990.

Dame Jane Goodall

Jane Goodall was born in London in 1934. She is one of the best known ethologists and primatologists (people who study primates). She studied at Cambridge University, and then worked with the anthropologist Louis Leakey and his wife Henrietta when they were searching for early human remains in Africa. Leakey was very impressed with Jane and asked her to study the chimpanzees of Gombe Stream National Park in Tanzania. She came back to England to complete her PhD, and from then on the focus of her work was Gombe.

Goodall's detailed observations of chimpanzee behaviour allowed scientists to build up a picture of the way individuals interact, and the way aggressive behaviour builds up and is dealt with. Her studies have helped move forward the boundaries of knowledge on both chimp and human behaviour. She is also actively involved in conservation work.

Find out more

Books

Fullick, Ann. *Life Science In Depth: Body Systems and Health* (Heinemann Library, 2006)

Green, Christopher. *New Toddler Taming* (Vermilion, 2006)

Cash, Adam. *Psychology for Dummies* (John Wiley & Sons, 2002)

Websites

http://news.bbc.co.uk/1/hi/health/medical_notes/473673.stm
Read about the dangers of smoking.

http://nobelprize.org/educational_games/medicine/pavlov/readmore.html
Find out all about the work of Pavlov and his dogs.

http://nobelprize.org/educational_games/medicine/split-brain
Play this game to help you understand how the different areas of your brain work.

www.nhsdirect.nhs.uk/articles/article.aspx?articleId=2344
Learn more about the health risks of smoking and ways to give up.

www.knowyourlimits.gov.uk
Discover lots of information on drinking and alcohol use and abuse. Play the game to find out whether you really know your limits when it comes to drinking.

www.rcpsych.ac.uk/mentalhealthinformation/mentalhealthandgrowingup/ 2goodparenting.aspx
Find out all about good parenting.

Topics for further study

Biruté Galdikas and her orang-utan studies.

Dian Fossey and her work with mountain gorillas.

Konrad Lorenz and his geese.

Sigmund Freud and psychoanalysis.

Harry Harlow and his baby rhesus monkeys.

The development of language in chimpanzees.

Piaget and his work on child development.

The Stanford Prison Experiment. This is a famous experiment on how people behave when they are put in a position of power and how they behave as prisoners. (www.prisonexp.org)

Ways to change behaviour for the better. Investigate ways to reduce or stop drinking or smoking. Find out which methods are the most successful and why.

Glossary

aggression   behaviour that intimidates, frightens, or hurts another animal or person

chromosome   structure found in all living cells that carries genetic information

conditioned reflexes   reflexes learned through repeating an action

contraception   prevention of sperm from meeting a fertile egg during sexual intercourse

correlation   linked relationship between two different factors

culture   shared system of beliefs, attitudes, and values of a group of people

DNA (deoxyribonucleic acid)   material that forms the genetic information in the cells

dominant   organism at the top of the social order in a group

ethical issues   issues in which there is an element of right and wrong, good or bad, which depends on the views of an individual or of society as a whole

ethologist   scientist who studies the behaviour of animals, particularly when they are in their natural environment

ethology   the study of animal behaviour, particularly in the natural environment

evaluate   assess the strengths and weaknesses of an investigation

gene   section of DNA that is the basic unit of inheritance

hierarchy   ranking of individuals in a social group or herd

hormone   chemical produced in the body that controls specific actions. Sex hormones control sexual development.

infertility   being unable to produce offspring

innate   behaviour that is pre-programmed and does not have to be learnt

instinct   behaviour that is pre-programmed and does not have to be learnt

longitudinal studies   series of observations carried out on the same people over many years

monoamine oxidase (MAOA)   chemical that breaks down chemical messages in the brain

MRI (magnetic resonance imaging) scanner   scanner that produces an image of the molecules that make up a substance. It is very useful for seeing the soft tissues of the human body such as the brain.

nerve impulse   electrical message that travels through the nervous system

neuroscientist   scientist who studies the nervous system

obese   very overweight, with a BMI of more than 30

pheromone   chemical produced by an animal that influences the behaviour or development of another animal of the same species

psychiatry   branch of medicine involving the treatment of mental health problems

psychology   study of the mind, based on behaviour

sense organ   organ that is sensitive to a stimulus such as sight, sound, or smell

sensitivity   awareness to a change in the environment

sexually transmitted diseases (STDs)   diseases that are passed from one person to another through sexual contact

stimulus   something that causes a response in a body part or organ, for example a pin prick or a sound

territory   area that an animal, pair of animals, or group of animals defends

Index